The Ultimate Secrets to Sustainable Weight Loss:

Achieve Your Goals, Transform Your Mindset, Habits, and Emotions through a Practical 30-Day Meal Plan

Dr. Michelle J. Salazar

Copyright

Copyright ©2024 by Dr. Michelle J. Salazar

Table of Contents

In order to help you achieve personal success and happiness, feel better physically, and have more energy and resilience, I wrote this book as a comprehensive guide to health management. I have observed frequently that our basic riches in life is our state of health. Improving your relationship with your body is one of the best strategies to get healthier. One of the best ways to attain excellent health is to understand how your body functions and live in harmony with its natural state. People genuinely want to lose fat when they talk about becoming younger or dropping weight. Additionally, there is a seemingly endless supply of knowledge regarding weight loss; however, not much of it goes beyond food and exercise.

Therefore this book is here to help you understand how your body works in relation to the amount of food you eat. This holistic method incorporates and integrates viewpoints from the physical, emotional, mental, and spiritual domains. I wrote this book to give you additional information about reaching your optimum weight and to help you find doable steps you may take to look and feel younger.

It's possible that you've been trying and failing to reduce weight. If that's the case, I think I know the solution. I believe you have been consuming incorrect foods. Research has demonstrated that eating the correct foods, such as nutrient-rich foods, can help you lose weight successfully instead of dieting, as many people believe. These foods are some of the slimmest, most fulfilling, and greatest foods for weight loss that you can find. Rather than being high in calories, they are high in vitamins, minerals, fiber, omega-3s, antioxidants, phytonutrients, and other nutrients that promote weight loss. You can shed pounds in a healthy way by trying out these Foods. This is the essence of this book.

This book will also show you how eating a diet high in nutrients can help you maintain your weight by reducing your intake of nutrient-poor foods, which are high in fat, salt, calories, and sugar and can induce weight gain. It's a novel, healthful method of weight loss. You'll discover the importance of nourishing your body with nutrient-rich, unprocessed foods and how it contributes to a healthy weight loss program. Foods that are high in nutrients for their calorie content are considered to be nutrient-rich.

Your body won't work effectively to reduce excess weight if you don't provide it the nutrition it needs to function. Additionally, you will experience weariness, tension, and exhaustion, which will deplete your motivation to keep going on your weight loss journey. By choosing tasty, nutrient-rich foods—like the World's Healthiest Foods—and cooking them in a way that both preserves and enhances their flavor.

And my effective 30-day meal plan for healthy weight loss will assist you in starting a pleasant, healthy lifestyle that will help you achieve your weight management objectives as well as your desire for vibrant health and energy. I wanted to design the greatest plan I could for you. You'll consume better and healthier things than you ever would have imagined with the help of this regimen. The Plan will teach you how to choose the proper foods, including high-energy vegetables, crisp salads, luscious fruits, high-fiber legumes, lean protein, and more. It will also help you improve your eating habits by emphasizing healthy fats and carbohydrates as well as loads of fiber. The focus of the book Healthy Weight Loss - Without Dieting is on achieving both weight loss and improved health.

By implementing new, healthy eating habits and engaging in regular exercise, this proven weight reduction strategy, The Healthiest Way of Eating, will provide you the power to take charge of your weight loss. If you decide to commit to losing weight, I think this book will help you achieve your desired level of well-being and a long, healthy life in addition to helping you lose weight in a healthy way by keeping you informed, strong, and healthy.

Introduction

A poor diet combined with little exercise is the root cause of many long-term issues. Without a doubt, our genetic makeup has a significant influence on our behavior and its outcomes. However, the places and people we live with are just as significant. Over the past ten years, the latter idea has gained more and more traction as we've learned that those who hang out with healthy friends—those who eat better and exercise more—are actually more likely to be in good health themselves. It is also true that those who are obese typically have acquaintances who are obese.

Successful behavior change is influenced by a wide range of factors, including barriers, attitudes, beliefs, and knowledge. Here, it's crucial to remember that information on its own is insufficient! Physician weight reduction counseling leads to clinically significant weight loss, according to a recent meta-analysis titled "Physician Weight Loss Advice and Patient Weight Loss Behavior Change." The majority of the studies included in the meta-analysis evaluated the effects of behavioral illnesses that affect people.

These habits have their origins deeply ingrained in a culture that has progressively reduced the amount of physical activity in our lives and increased access to high-fat, high-calorie foods. This combination has been lethal for our community. In comparison to people with good cardiorespiratory fitness, those with low aerobic fitness—a result of a sedentary lifestyle—have a 56% greater risk of heart disease and a 35% increased chance of Alzheimer's dementia. One in ten deaths globally are thought to be caused by physical inactivity; if this factor could be decreased by just 25%, 1.3 million lives could be prevented annually. Similarly, diets high in saturated fat have been linked to increased incidence of heart disease.

Given the strong evidence, attempts to reverse the obesity trend must take into account social networks, the environment, biology, and, finally, behavior. Why does our society continue to battle with unhealthy eating habits and insufficient physical activity, given the risks associated with both behaviors and the advantages of adhering to prescribed recommendations for both? This inquiry has a lengthy and intricate response.

It is important to note, therefore, that even a small amount of weight loss can have a significant effect on health outcomes. It's not necessary to shed fifty to one hundred pounds to noticeably lower one's risk of illness. For instance, the Diabetes Prevention Program discovered that a person's risk of acquiring diabetes can be considerably decreased by losing merely 7% of their body weight, or 17.5 pounds for a 250-pound individual. Obesity and obstructive sleep apnea are also linked conditions. There is a 3% reduction in the risk of obstructive sleep apnea for every 1% drop in weight. One of the most common long-term medical disorders is osteoarthritis.

Chapter 1

A successful weight loss lies within you

Starting the process of weight loss often involves trying out different diets like Weight Watchers, Atkins, South Beach, or those favored by celebrities. Many people eagerly devour magazines for tips on shedding pounds, drawn to promises of rapid weight loss. While you may have experienced success in losing weight with these diets, the likelihood of regaining it, and perhaps even gaining extra pounds, is high. The key to achieving lasting success in weight loss lies within understanding and addressing internal factors. These factors are inside of you and what you can handle. It all depends on your level of discipline.

Therefore, to truly succeed in your weight loss endeavors, it's essential to focus on the internal aspects of your journey. This is because, rather than solely relying on external diet plans, shifting your perspective to an internal approach can yield more sustainable results. This involves delving into the mindset, habits, and emotional aspects related to eating and lifestyle choices.

How Your Mindset, Habits, Emotions can Give You the Desired Weight Loss You Want

One fundamental aspect of weight loss is understanding your mindset toward food. Instead of viewing food as a mere source of calories, explore your relationship with it. Are you eating for nourishment, emotional comfort, or out of habit? Identifying and addressing these psychological aspects can pave the way for a healthier relationship with food. Habits play a crucial role in weight management. Assessing your daily routines and identifying unhealthy habits can be transformative. Simple changes, such as incorporating regular physical activity or opting for nutritious snacks, can contribute significantly to your weight loss journey.

Emotional factors also play a significant role in weight gain and loss. Stress, boredom, and emotional triggers can lead to overeating or making unhealthy food choices. Developing coping mechanisms that don't involve food, such as exercise, meditation, or hobbies, can contribute to a more balanced emotional state.

Furthermore, understanding your body's signals is vital. Pay attention to hunger and fullness cues, and eat mindfully. Recognizing when you're genuinely hungry versus eating out of boredom or stress can prevent unnecessary calorie consumption. A holistic approach involves cultivating a positive relationship with your body. Rather than focusing solely on appearance or societal expectations, prioritize overall well-being. Celebrate small victories, whether they are improvements in energy levels, mood, or overall health.

The path to successful weight loss extends beyond external diets and quick fixes. By turning inward and addressing internal factors like mindset, habits, emotions, and body signals, you can create lasting and positive changes. Developing a holistic understanding of your relationship with food and your body sets the foundation for a healthier and more sustainable weight loss journey.

Weight Loss Diet Problems

The idea that you've failed at dieting might be a message you've heard, but a more precise perspective suggests that it's the weight loss diet that has let you down. Many diets emphasize quick fixes, leading to temporary weight loss, but they often neglect the root causes that contribute to weight gain in the first place. In simpler terms, these diets only address the surface, overlooking what's happening on the inside.

When we talk about weight loss diet failure, it's crucial to understand that it's not about your personal failure. The blame lies with the limitations of many popular diets that promise swift results without addressing the deeper issues. Most of these diets concentrate on external changes, like eating less or following a specific meal plan, without delving into the reasons behind your weight gain.

For instance, you embark on a diet, restrict your food intake, maybe even lose a few pounds initially, and feel a sense of accomplishment. However, more often than not, this weight loss is short-lived. The real challenge surfaces when you realize the pounds start creeping back, and sometimes even more than before. This frustrating cycle is a common experience for many who have tried popular diets.

The inherent problem with these diets is their focus on short-term fixes. They might help you shed weight quickly, but they lack a sustainable approach. Why? Because they don't address the root causes that contribute to your weight concerns. It's like putting a band-aid on a wound without addressing the underlying infection – the problem persists.

Let's break down the flaws in many weight loss diets. They often center around external changes, such as altering your eating habits or following a specific exercise routine. While these changes can lead to initial weight loss, they don't address the internal factors that influence your weight. Factors like your relationship with food, emotional triggers, and lifestyle habits are crucial components that these diets overlook.

The "outside" changes promoted by these diets might give a temporary illusion of success, but they miss the mark when it comes to achieving lasting and meaningful weight loss. To truly succeed in your weight loss journey, it's essential to shift the focus from external changes to internal understanding.

Understanding the internal factors involves a more profound exploration of your relationship with food. Are you eating out of boredom, stress, or genuine hunger? Identifying these emotional triggers is a vital step in establishing a healthier connection with food. It's not just about what you eat but also why and how you eat.

Habits play a pivotal role in the weight loss equation. Many diets emphasize specific meal plans or exercise routines, but they often neglect to address your daily habits. Simple adjustments, like incorporating regular physical activity or choosing nutritious snacks, can significantly impact your weight loss journey.

Emotional well-being is another internal factor that should not be overlooked. Stress, boredom, or emotional upheavals can lead to unhealthy eating patterns. Developing alternative coping mechanisms, such as practicing mindfulness, engaging in hobbies, or seeking support, can contribute to a more balanced emotional state.

Moreover, paying attention to your body's signals is crucial. Many diets impose strict rules that may not align with your body's natural cues of hunger and fullness. Practicing mindful eating, listening to your body, and distinguishing between genuine hunger and emotional cravings can prevent unnecessary calorie consumption.

In essence, the path to successful weight loss goes beyond mere external changes. It involves a holistic understanding of your internal landscape, addressing factors like mindset, habits, emotions, and bodily signals. Shifting from a focus on quick fixes to a sustainable, internal approach lays the foundation for lasting success in your weight loss journey. It's not about blaming yourself for diet failures but recognizing the need for a more comprehensive and enduring strategy.

Where Success Lies in Weight Loss

The journey to weight loss demands more than just shedding pounds; it requires a transformative exploration of the latent powers within you. In other words, a guide is essential to illuminate this path, leading you to the discovery of the profound control you possess. The journey encompasses not only physical aspects but delves into the realms of mental, emotional, and social powers, essential elements often overlooked in the pursuit of fitting into those elusive jeans once again.

Contrary to misleading messages that suggest your worth is solely defined by control over your eating habits, the truth is that every person possesses a reservoir of magnificence. It is a wellspring of mental prowess, emotional resilience, social grace, and physical strength.

These powers lie dormant, waiting to be harnessed to achieve the life you aspire to lead.

The first step toward sustainable weight loss involves healing past wounds. These wounds, whether rooted in emotional struggles or past setbacks, can act as barriers preventing you from realizing your full potential. By addressing and overcoming these obstacles, you pave the way for a foundation that goes beyond mere weight loss—it becomes a platform for personal empowerment.

Recognizing the inherent power within you is not just about shedding pounds; it's a holistic approach to self-discovery and self-empowerment. As you navigate the journey, guided by a mentor, you unravel the layers of your psyche, tapping into the mental reserves that contribute to your overall well-being.

Moreover, your emotional resilience plays a pivotal role in this process. Understanding and managing emotions associated with food and self-image are crucial steps toward achieving lasting change. Social powers, too, are significant; a supportive network can provide encouragement and strength as you navigate the challenges of reshaping your lifestyle.

Physical power is not merely about the capability to exercise but extends to cultivating a healthy relationship with your body. Recognizing its signals, providing nourishment, and embracing physical activity become integral components of your newfound journey toward holistic well-being. Turning failure into success in the realm of weight loss involves a profound shift in perspective. It transcends the superficial pursuit of fitting into clothes and delves into the depths of your being. By acknowledging and cultivating your mental, emotional, social, and physical powers, you not only shed weight but also lay the groundwork for a life of enduring success and fulfillment.

The Practical Aspect of Weight Loss

If the mere thought of a weight loss diet feels like a burden, success might remain elusive. Conversely, by embracing an empowering program that seamlessly integrates into your lifestyle while adding an element of enjoyment, you unlock the doors to triumph. Therefore, shedding a whole size in just two weeks becomes not just a possibility but a tangible reality. The so-called "secret" lies in the fusion of a well-tested exercise regimen and a synergistic eating plan, both grounded in simplicity, clarity, and practicality.

The foundation of a successful weight loss strategy is an exercise program that goes beyond being a routine; it becomes a lifestyle companion. The key is to choose a program that aligns effortlessly with your daily life, ensuring that it's not a source of stress but a catalyst for positive change. Simplicity is paramount; intricate routines may discourage consistency. By incorporating manageable exercises that seamlessly blend into your routine, you create a sustainable approach that stands the test of time.

Clarity is the beacon that guides your fitness journey. Understanding the purpose and benefits of each exercise fosters a deeper connection between your efforts and results. This clarity serves as a motivating force, transforming workouts from mere tasks into meaningful steps towards your well-defined goals.

Practicality acts as the linchpin, holding together the various components of your weight loss plan. It involves choosing exercises and activities that cater to your lifestyle, making it easier to stay committed. A program that requires minimal equipment and can be done in the comfort of your home or local surroundings ensures that practicality remains at the forefront.

Complementing your exercise plan, an eating strategy is crucial for holistic success. It's not about restrictive diets that leave you feeling deprived; instead, it's about adopting a plan that harmonizes with your newfound sense of personal power. The inner work you've done to embrace this power becomes the bedrock upon which your eating plan is built. Together, they form a dynamic duo that propels you toward lasting change.

Guidance is pivotal in navigating this transformative journey. With the right mentor, you transcend the limitations of conventional weight loss diets. It's not just about shedding pounds; it's about achieving victory in every facet of your life. This holistic approach ensures that your outer beauty aligns harmoniously with your inner beauty, creating a comprehensive transformation that radiates from within.

Chapter 2

Simple Steps for Losing Weight

A lot of people in Australia are dealing with a big problem called obesity. It's like a health crisis. Many companies sell pills and stuff promising quick weight loss, but most of the time, these don't really help. The same goes for diets – there are so many, and it's hard to know which ones work. What we really need are some easy and proven tips that anyone can follow, no matter how they are right now. Let's get into it.

- **Drink More Water:**

Ensuring an adequate water intake is a fundamental and straightforward approach to improving overall well-being. In Australia, a significant number of people fall short in their daily water consumption, and this has profound effects on the body's functionality. The impact goes beyond simple thirst; it disrupts the body's ability to efficiently eliminate toxins and waste.

When we don't drink enough water, our bodies enter a perpetual state of thirst. This not only leads to discomfort but also hampers the body's natural detoxification processes. Think of water as the cleansing agent that helps flush out the bad stuff from our systems. Without sufficient water, these impurities linger, potentially causing various health issues.

Moreover, dehydration can affect our energy levels and cognitive functions. Even mild dehydration can lead to feelings of fatigue and difficulty concentrating. By ensuring an adequate water supply, we support our body's ability to carry out essential functions, promoting physical and mental well-being.

In practical terms, making a conscious effort to drink more water throughout the day can be a game-changer. Starting the day with a glass of water and keeping a water bottle handy are simple habits that can have a significant impact. This isn't about following a complex regimen; it's about incorporating a basic yet powerful practice into our daily lives.

The benefits of proper hydration extend beyond weight loss; it contributes to improved digestion, clearer skin, and enhanced overall vitality. In the pursuit of a healthier lifestyle, prioritizing water intake is a foundational step. It's not just a remedy for thirst; it's a vital component for the efficient functioning of our bodies, ensuring we are better equipped to tackle the challenges of daily life.

- **Eat More Often, But Less:**

Shedding those extra pounds often comes with the misconception that it requires strict deprivation and eating less. However, the reality is more nuanced – an approach centered around consistent, smaller meals can be a key to successful and sustainable weight loss.

The analogy of a burning fire aptly captures the essence of this strategy. Imagine your metabolism as that fire – it needs a constant supply of fuel to keep burning efficiently. Eating regularly, even if the meals are smaller, keeps the metabolic fire alive, preventing it from dwindling and slowing down. In simpler terms, it's about maintaining a steady flow of energy to keep the body's calorie-burning process in full swing.Skipping meals, particularly breakfast, is often seen as a shortcut to weight loss, but it can have counterproductive effects. Our bodies are smart; when faced with prolonged periods without food, they enter a sort of survival mode. This slows down the metabolism, making it more challenging to burn calories efficiently. It's like letting the fire go out, and reigniting it becomes a tougher task.

Losing weight doesn't mean we have to go hungry. Instead, it involves a strategic approach of eating smaller meals more frequently. This method ensures that our metabolism stays active, consistently burning calories throughout the day. Starting the day with breakfast is like giving the metabolic fire a kickstart – it sets the tone for the rest of the day.

The concept of smaller, more frequent meals isn't about drastically reducing the amount of food we eat. It's about distributing our daily calorie intake across several meals, preventing energy highs and lows. This approach helps in avoiding overeating during main meals and keeps our metabolism humming along steadily.

Incorporating breakfast into our daily routine is a critical aspect of this strategy. The morning meal provides the body with the essential fuel it needs after the overnight fast. Even if it's a quick drink and a piece of fruit, it jumpstarts our metabolism, signaling to our body that it's time to get into calorie-burning mode. Essentially, breakfast acts as the ignition for the metabolic engine, setting it in motion for the day ahead.

Moreover, eating smaller, well-balanced meals throughout the day helps regulate blood sugar levels. This prevents extreme spikes and crashes, reducing the likelihood of intense hunger that often leads to unhealthy food choices. It's a holistic approach that not only aids in weight loss but also promotes overall health and well-being. The strategy of eating smaller, more frequent meals is a practical and sustainable approach to weight loss. It aligns with the body's natural processes, keeping the metabolic fire burning consistently. It's not about deprivation or extreme measures; it's about nourishing our bodies smartly to achieve lasting results. So, let's shift our focus from eating less to eating right, ensuring that our metabolic fire stays alive and well on the path to a healthier lifestyle.

- **Move Around More:**

In the pursuit of weight loss, the notion of rigorous exercise regimens can be intimidating and discouraging. The good news is that shedding those extra pounds doesn't necessitate running marathons or enduring grueling workouts. Instead, a simpler and more enjoyable approach involves incorporating more movement into our daily lives. The essence of this strategy is beautifully encapsulated in the idea that we don't need to run marathons to lose weight. The emphasis is on making small but significant changes in our daily routines to enhance physical activity. It's about embracing movement as a lifestyle, not just a chore reserved for the gym.

Taking the stairs instead of the elevator is a prime example of how effortless adjustments can contribute to increased daily activity. This simple choice not only burns calories but also strengthens leg muscles and boosts cardiovascular health. It's a small change that, when made consistently, adds up to significant positive effects on our overall well-being.

Walking a bit more is another accessible way to boost daily activity levels. Whether it's opting for a longer route to the grocery store or taking a stroll during a lunch break, incorporating more steps into our day is a practical and achievable goal. The cumulative impact of these extra steps contributes to a higher calorie expenditure, supporting weight loss in a sustainable manner.

Playful interactions, such as engaging with kids or incorporating dance into daily routines, exemplify the joyous aspect of increased movement. It's a reminder that exercise doesn't have to be a serious, regimented activity; it can be fun and enjoyable. Dancing to favorite tunes not only burns calories but also lifts spirits, making it a dual-purpose activity that aligns with the goal of weight loss while promoting mental well-being.

Explained Simply: The crux of this approach is that hardcore exercises are not a prerequisite for weight loss. Instead, it involves incorporating simple and enjoyable activities into our daily lives. Taking the stairs, going for a walk, playing with kids, or dancing are all accessible ways to move more without the need for elaborate workout routines.

The key to success lies in making these activities enjoyable. When movement is fun, it becomes a sustainable part of our routine. It's not about adhering to a strict exercise regimen that feels like a burden; it's about finding pleasure in the process. This mindset shift is crucial in fostering a positive relationship with physical activity, ensuring that it becomes a natural and enjoyable aspect of our daily lives.

Moreover, embracing movement as a lifestyle choice goes beyond the immediate goal of weight loss. It contributes to overall health, improving cardiovascular fitness, enhancing muscle tone, and boosting mood. It's a holistic approach that recognizes the interconnectedness of physical and mental well-being.

The message is clear: we don't need extreme workouts to achieve weight loss. Simple, enjoyable movements incorporated into our daily routines can make a significant difference. Taking the stairs, going for a walk, playing with kids, or dancing are all valid and accessible ways to enhance physical activity. Let's shift our perspective from exercise as a chore to movement as a joyous and integral part of a healthier lifestyle.

- **Know Why You Want to Lose Weight:**

A lot people do not know why they want to lose weight. Understanding the underlying reasons for embarking on a weight loss journey is a fundamental and powerful aspect of the process. The "Why" behind our efforts serves as a guiding force, providing motivation and resilience when faced with challenges. Whether driven by health concerns, a desire for increased self-esteem, or the wish to be present for loved ones, having a clear and compelling reason can make all the difference on the road to weight loss success.

The importance of knowing why we want to lose weight cannot be overstated. It serves as a beacon that illuminates the path ahead, offering a sense of purpose and direction. When the journey becomes challenging, as it inevitably does, this intrinsic motivation becomes the driving force that keeps us moving forward.

For many individuals, the "Why" is intricately linked to health. The desire to lead a healthier lifestyle, prevent potential health issues, or improve existing conditions can be a powerful motivator. Recognizing that weight loss is not just about appearance but also about enhancing overall well-being creates a more holistic and sustainable approach.

Imagine your "Why" as a big reason to keep going. It's the fuel that keeps your engine running on the tougher days. Maybe you want to be healthier or feel better about yourself – whatever it is, having a strong "Why" is like having a powerful motivator in your corner.

Self-esteem and body image are also common driving factors. Wanting to feel more confident and comfortable in one's own skin is a valid and impactful reason to pursue weight loss. The emotional benefits that come with an improved self-image contribute significantly to mental well-being, creating a positive feedback loop. Being there for loved ones is another poignant "Why." Whether it's wanting to actively engage with children or be a supportive partner, the motivation to enhance one's ability to participate fully in the lives of loved ones is a powerful catalyst for change. This external focus on relationships underscores the interconnectedness between personal health and the well-being of those we care about.

Having a strong "Why" is particularly crucial during challenging times. Weight loss journeys are seldom linear; they come with ups and downs. In moments of difficulty, the clarity of our motivation becomes a source of resilience. It's the reminder of the bigger picture, the overarching goal that extends beyond immediate obstacles.

In essence, the "Why" is the anchor that grounds us in our weight loss journey. It transforms the process from a mere pursuit of physical changes to a profound and meaningful personal transformation. The strength of this motivation lies in its personal nature – it's unique to each individual and reflects their values, aspirations, and priorities.

Therefore, knowing why we want to lose weight is akin to having a powerful reason that keeps us going. Whether it's for health, self-esteem, or loved ones, this intrinsic motivation acts as a steady force during the inevitable challenges. It's a reminder that the journey is not just about shedding pounds; it's about embracing a healthier and more fulfilling life.

Lastly, losing weight doesn't have to be complicated. These simple tips – drinking more water, eating regularly but in smaller portions, moving around more, and knowing why we want to lose weight – can work for anyone. It's not just about looking good; it's about feeling better and being healthier. Let's make it simple and achievable for everyone.

Chapter 3

Overcoming Weight Loss Plateaus: 5 Practical Tips for Success

If you find yourself stuck in a weight loss plateau, where your body seems resistant to shedding those last few pounds despite maintaining your diet and exercise routine, fret not. Plateaus are common, and with a few strategic adjustments, you can kickstart your weight loss journey again. In this comprehensive guide, we will explore five easy tips to overcome weight loss plateaus and get your body back on the path to success.

- **Change Your Calorie Intake:**

Calorie manipulation is a potent tool to break through a weight loss plateau. Begin by closely monitoring your daily calorie intake and consider making slight reductions. This gradual adjustment can signal to your body that change is happening, prompting it to respond by shedding excess weight.

An alternative approach is the zigzag method, where you cycle between days of reduced and increased calorie intake. This fluctuation prevents your body from settling into a comfort zone and encourages it to adapt to varying energy levels. Remember to make minor adjustments and closely monitor your weight with each change to ensure a sustainable and healthy progression.

- **Replace a Snack or Two:**

A simple yet effective strategy is to rethink your snack choices. If you tend to indulge in sugary or high-calorie snacks, consider replacing them with healthier alternatives. Opt for fruits like apples and bananas, or vegetables like carrots and celery paired with a low-fat dip. Not only are these options filling, but they also contribute to healthy weight loss. This adjustment not only addresses your caloric intake but also enhances the nutritional value of your diet.

- **Extend Your Exercise Routine:**

Physical activity plays a crucial role in weight loss, and sometimes all it takes is a bit more time dedicated to exercise. If you've hit a plateau, consider extending your daily workout duration. If you typically exercise for 30 minutes, push yourself to 45 minutes.

Incorporating non-strenuous activities like walking into your routine is an excellent way to boost calorie expenditure. Simple adjustments, such as parking farther from your destination or taking short walks during breaks, can significantly impact your weight loss efforts.

- **Monitor Your Nutrient Intake:**

What you eat matters just as much as how much you eat. Evaluate your diet to ensure a balanced intake of nutrients. If your diet leans heavily towards sugars and carbohydrates, consider incorporating more protein-rich foods. Protein is known for its fat-burning properties and its ability to provide sustained energy. Protein-rich snacks, like protein bars, can be convenient options to enhance your daily intake. Additionally, ensure you're getting an adequate amount of water and fiber, addressing potential deficiencies in these areas.

- **Opt for Smaller, More Frequent Meals:**

Breaking away from the traditional three large meals a day can be a game-changer. Instead, experiment with smaller, more frequent meals throughout the day. Reduce portion sizes during regular meals and introduce healthy snacks between meals. This approach not only helps in boosting metabolism but also prevents excessive hunger, reducing the likelihood of overeating during main meals. Striking this balance contributes to a sustainable and healthier approach to weight loss.

Weight loss plateaus are a common roadblock on the journey to a healthier you. The key to overcoming these plateaus lies in making strategic and sustainable adjustments to your lifestyle. Whether it's modifying your calorie intake, choosing healthier snacks, extending your exercise routine, optimizing nutrient intake, or adjusting your meal frequency, these tips provide a roadmap for breaking through plateaus and reigniting your weight loss journey.

Remember, the goal is not rapid weight loss, but rather a sustainable and healthy progression towards your long-term goals. Use these practical tips to overcome your plateau, embrace a healthier lifestyle, and achieve the weight loss success you desire. Your journey to a better you starts today.

Chapter 4

Choosing the Right Weight Loss Plan

In the quest for shedding those extra kilograms, the abundance of weight loss plans can be overwhelming, leaving many individuals feeling fatigued and unsure of where to begin. Whether you're aiming to lose a modest amount or embark on a more substantial weight loss journey, selecting the right plan is a critical decision that should align with your lifestyle and individual needs. In this chapter, we will explore the key considerations for choosing a weight loss plan, ensuring that it not only aids in achieving your goals but also becomes an integral and sustainable part of your daily routine.

- **Understanding Your Style**:

The first step in selecting an effective weight loss plan is understanding your unique style and preferences. What works seamlessly for one person may not be the ideal fit for another. It's crucial to assess your daily routine, identify the types of foods you enjoy, and acknowledge your body's specific requirements.

- **Dietary Preferences**:

Consider your culinary preferences. Do you have a sweet tooth, or do you lean towards savory delights?

Evaluate if you have specific dietary restrictions or preferences, such as vegetarianism or a low-carb approach.

- **Eating Habits:**

Reflect on your typical eating pattern. Do you prefer three square meals a day, or do you find satisfaction in smaller, more frequent meals?

By aligning your weight loss plan with your style, you enhance the likelihood of adherence, making the journey more enjoyable and sustainable.

- **Studying the Risks:**

Not all weight loss plans are created equal, and some carry inherent risks that can impact both your progress and overall health. It's essential to conduct a thorough examination of potential risks associated with different plans.

- **Pace of Weight Loss:**

Rapid weight loss may seem enticing, but it can be detrimental to your body, especially if sustained over an extended period. Consider the health implications and opt for gradual progress to ensure sustainability.

- **Weight Loss Pills:**

Exercise caution with weight loss pills. These can pose risks if taken without proper medical supervision. Consult with your physician before incorporating any supplements into your regimen.

- **Health Conditions:**

Take into account any existing health conditions you may have. Certain diets may exacerbate pre-existing problems. For instance, a meat-centric diet might not be suitable if you have digestive or heart issues.

- **Medications**:

If you are on prescription medications or have significant health concerns, consult your doctor before embarking on a weight loss plan. Your health professional can provide valuable insights and tailor recommendations based on your individual circumstances.

- **Tailoring to Your Lifestyle:**

A successful weight loss plan seamlessly integrates into your lifestyle, becoming a natural extension of your daily routine. Consider the practical aspects that can contribute to the plan's long-term viability.

Realistic Meal Plans:

Opt for a plan that offers realistic and sustainable meal plans. Extreme diets often lead to short-term success but are challenging to maintain over time.

Flexibility:

Look for flexibility in your chosen plan. Life is dynamic, and your weight loss journey should accommodate occasional deviations without inducing guilt or derailing progress.

Long-Term Commitment:

Evaluate your commitment level. Choose a plan that aligns with your readiness for long-term lifestyle changes rather than quick fixes.

Professional Guidance:

If uncertainty persists or if you have specific health concerns, seeking professional guidance is paramount. Consulting with a nutritionist, dietitian, or healthcare professional can provide tailored advice and ensure that your chosen weight loss plan is safe and effective for your unique circumstances.

- **Personalizing Your Approach**:

A one-size-fits-all approach seldom yields optimal results in weight loss. Personalization is key. Consider working with a professional to develop a plan tailored to your preferences, goals, and health considerations.

Choosing a weight loss plan is a pivotal decision that goes beyond shedding kilograms; it's about cultivating a healthier, more sustainable lifestyle. By understanding your style, studying potential risks, tailoring to your lifestyle, seeking professional guidance, and personalizing your approach, you empower yourself to make informed decisions on this transformative journey.

Remember, the path to weight loss is not a sprint but a marathon. Select a plan that aligns with your individuality, embraces gradual progress, and positions you for long-term success. This comprehensive guide serves as your compass, guiding you towards a weight loss plan that not only meets your goals but enriches your life along the way.

Chapter 5

Types of Weight Loss Diets

The key to having a successful weight loss lies in understanding each type of weight loss diet, evaluating its impact on your body, and aligning it with your lifestyle. The weight loss diets include:

Diets for Fast Weight Loss:

Fast weight loss diets are designed for those seeking quick results. While not recommended for long-term sustainability, they can provide a rapid initial reduction in weight.

Examples include low-carb diets, three-to-five-day meal replacement shakes, water or juice fasts, and alternate vegetable/fruit diets.

Considerations:

- These diets offer a quick fix but may be challenging and possibly unhealthy for prolonged use.
- Not suitable for sustained, long-term weight management.

Low Calorie Weight Loss Diets:

Low calorie diets involve reducing daily calorie intake to promote weight loss. Monitoring calories can be done through food labels, calorie guides, or programs like Weight Watchers, which uses a point system based on calories, fiber, and fat grams.

Considerations:

- Effective for gradual weight loss.
- Requires meticulous calorie tracking.

- Weight Watchers offers a structured approach with a point system.

Fixed Menu Plans::

Fixed menu plans provide a pre-determined list of foods based on individual preferences and needs. Simplifies meal planning during the weight loss phase.

Considerations:

- While convenient, learning to plan meals independently is essential for long-term success.
- Helps establish structure but necessitates transitioning to self-planned meals post-diet.

Exchange Food Diet:

An exchange food diet involves planning meals with servings from various food groups based on calorie intake. Allows flexibility in food choices within specified calorie limits.

Considerations:

- Ideal for a post-fixed menu diet as it provides autonomy in food selection.
- Encourages a balanced intake across different food groups.

Low Fat Diet:

Low fat diets aim to reduce overall fat intake, especially saturated fats, in alignment with the food pyramid. Approximately 30% of daily calories should come from fats.

Considerations:

- Promotes healthy weight loss and heart health.
- Requires careful scrutiny as some "low-fat" foods can be high in sugar.

- Encourages choosing healthier options and limiting saturated fats.

Weight Loss through Reduced Portions:

This approach focuses on reducing portion sizes while allowing flexibility in food choices.

Emphasizes eating slowly until satisfied but not overly full.

Considerations:

- Provides freedom in food selection but limits portion sizes.
- Encourages mindful eating and listening to hunger cues.

Pre-Packaged Meals and Formulas:

Utilizes pre-packaged meals and formulas designed for specific calorie intake and nutritional balance. Simplifies meal planning with ready-to-consume options.

Considerations:

- Offers convenience but may limit flexibility in food choices.
- Effective if adherence to prescribed meals is maintained.

It is very important to say that there is no one-size-fits-all solution for weight loss. Each type offers unique benefits and considerations, and the effectiveness of a plan depends on individual preferences, lifestyle, and health conditions. As you explore these varied approaches, remember that sustainable weight loss involves not just shedding kilograms but cultivating lasting lifestyle changes.

Therefore, before embarking on any weight loss plan, it's crucial to consult with your healthcare provider, especially if you have existing health conditions or are on medication. By combining knowledge, professional guidance, and a personalized approach, you can embark on a weight loss journey that aligns with your goals and sets the stage for a healthier, more fulfilling life.

Chapter 6

Boost Metabolism and Achieve Weight Loss through Smart Eating

The age-old adage "breakfast is the most important meal of the day" has received a powerful affirmation through recent research, shedding light on the significant impact of morning dietary choices on overall health. Beyond being a mere ritual, breakfast holds the key to enhancing metabolism and facilitating weight loss.

Breakfast Habits and Body Mass Index (BMI):

The National Heart, Lung, and Blood Institute in the US conducted a decade-long study involving 2,300 teenage girls, revealing a compelling correlation between breakfast habits and Body Mass Index (BMI). The study underscored that irrespective of physical activity levels, consuming high-fiber cereal at least three times a week significantly contributes to maintaining a lower BMI.

What You Should Know:

- High-fiber cereal emerged as a pivotal breakfast choice for weight management.
- The study challenges the misconception that skipping breakfast aids in calorie reduction.

- Regular breakfast consumption showcases long-term benefits in BMI regulation.

The Pitfalls of Skipping Breakfast:

Caloric Intake and Snacking Patterns:

While some individuals skip breakfast in an attempt to curtail overall calorie intake, this approach may backfire.

Breakfast deprivation often leads to increased snacking on unhealthy options like chocolate later in the day.

Performance and Fatigue:

Breakfast, even if a simple smoothie or a couple of pieces of fruit, plays a crucial role in enhancing work performance and reducing fatigue. The nutritional value derived from breakfast sustains energy levels throughout the day.

Beyond Caloric Intake:

Smart Food Choices:

Focusing not only on overall calorie intake but also on the quality of foods is paramount.

Opting for nutrient-dense choices like carrots over conventional breakfast items ensures a balance of fiber, phytochemicals, and essential vitamins.

Fruit Street Vendor vs. Muffin:

A strategic visit to a local fruit street vendor before work trumps opting for a nutritionally lacking muffin at a coffee shop. Investing in fresh fruits and vegetables yields both nutritional and long-term health benefits.

Debunking Caloric Restriction Myths:

Recent research dispels the notion that extreme caloric restriction, though extending the lifespan of mice by up to 50%, translates to similar outcomes in humans. For humans, the impact of a low-calorie diet might only extend life by a modest 7%.

Physiological Impact of Breakfast:

Contrary to calorie-restriction approaches, having breakfast is proven to physiologically boost metabolism. The metabolic enhancement achieved through breakfast consumption provides a cost-effective alternative to investing in diet pills.

Strategies for Boosting Metabolism:

- Incorporate high-fiber cereals, smoothies, or fresh fruit into your morning routine to kickstart metabolism.
- Consider a variety of nutrient-dense options, such as carrots, to diversify your breakfast choices.

Local Fruit Vendor Advantage:

Embrace the convenience of purchasing fresh fruits and vegetables from local vendors, making healthier choices more accessible than indulging in muffins or other less nutritious alternatives.

Mindful Eating Habits:

Cultivate a habit of mindful eating, listening to hunger cues, and choosing breakfast options that align with both nutritional needs and taste preferences.

The Holistic Approach to Weight Loss:

Recognize breakfast not merely as a standalone meal but as an integral part of a holistic lifestyle.

Embrace the long-term benefits of consistent breakfast habits for sustained weight management.

The breakfast paradigm transcends conventional wisdom, emerging as a potent catalyst for weight loss and metabolic enhancement. The findings from the National Heart, Lung, and Blood Institute's extensive study echo the sentiment that breakfast, particularly when rich in fiber, holds the key to maintaining a lower BMI.

By adopting smart eating habits, making strategic breakfast choices, and debunking myths surrounding extreme caloric restriction, individuals can embark on a journey of sustainable weight management. The breakfast table becomes a canvas for crafting a healthier, more energized, and metabolically boosted version of oneself. As you navigate the nuances of breakfast choices, remember that a well-informed approach to eating can be a transformative force in your quest for a balanced and vibrant life.

Chapter 7

Weight Loss Tips for Parents and Expecting Mothers

Parenthood and the journey to motherhood bring profound joy and responsibility, and for many, it sparks a desire to prioritize health. In this exploration, we delve into weight loss tips tailored for parents and expecting mothers. Early research sheds light on the impact of maternal eating habits on childhood weight, while the influence of sedentary activities in children underscores the importance of fostering a healthy lifestyle from an early age. Beyond these insights, we'll uncover the significance of variety in dietary choices, the pitfalls of unhealthy food patterns, and the benefits of incorporating raw fruits and vegetables into one's diet.

Maternal Eating Habits and Childhood Weight:

Early research suggests a link between maternal overeating during pregnancy and a higher likelihood of toddlers being overweight. Notable examples, such as Britney Spears, highlight the potential impact of maternal eating habits on childhood weight.

Impact on Food Habits:

Children exposed to maternal overeating may develop food-related challenges from a young age.Understanding the long-term consequences emphasizes the need for mindful eating habits during pregnancy.

Sedentary Activities and Childhood Obesity:

Challenges in Modern Lifestyles:

Sedentary activities, including excessive gaming and prolonged television watching, contribute to poor eating habits in children and teenagers.

The combination of sedentary behavior and unhealthy eating patterns increases the risk of childhood obesity evolving into adulthood.

Promoting Active Lifestyles:

Encouraging non-athletic activities, such as part-time jobs or school clubs, fosters a balanced and active lifestyle.

Limiting screen time and promoting outdoor play can mitigate the negative effects of sedentary activities.

Embracing Dietary Variety:

The Importance of Variety:

- Breaking free from food ruts and monotonous diets is essential for sustained health.
- Incorporating a variety of foods ensures a well-rounded nutrient intake and supports diverse health goals.

Planning Ahead:

Planning meals in advance and conducting research on diverse and healthy recipes helps avoid unhealthy food choices driven by convenience.

The Benefits of Raw Fruits and Vegetables:

Nutrient-Rich Choices:

- Consuming fruits and vegetables in their raw form preserves vital vitamins that can be diminished by cooking processes.
- Raw fruits and vegetables contribute enzymes beneficial for digestion, enhancing nutrient absorption.

Watermelon: A Nutrient Powerhouse:

Watermelon, rich in vitamin C, stands out as a nutritional powerhouse.

Lycopene, an effective antioxidant present in watermelon, offers additional health benefits, aligning it with other sources like tomatoes, red grapefruit, and guava.

Strategies for Integrating Changes:
Mindful Eating Practices:

- Developing mindfulness around eating habits during pregnancy and parenthood promotes healthier choices.

- Being conscious of portion sizes and savoring each bite can contribute to overall well-being.

Family-Friendly Recipes:

Exploring and creating family-friendly recipes that prioritize nutritional value ensures that health-conscious choices become an integral part of family life.

Cultivating a Healthy Family Environment:

Parents serve as role models, and adopting a healthy lifestyle sets the foundation for children.

Involving the whole family in physical activities and meal planning fosters a supportive environment.

Educational Initiatives:

Educating children about the benefits of a balanced diet and an active lifestyle empowers them to make informed choices.

Professional Guidance and Support:

- Consultation with Healthcare Providers:
- Expecting mothers should consult healthcare providers to tailor dietary choices to individual needs during pregnancy.
- Seeking guidance from nutritionists or healthcare professionals ensures a well-rounded approach to health.

The early influences of maternal eating habits on childhood weight and the pitfalls of sedentary activities in children underscore the need for intentional lifestyle choices. Embracing variety in dietary choices, incorporating raw fruits and vegetables, and cultivating mindful eating practices create a foundation for a healthy family environment.

As parents and expecting mothers navigate the complexities of nurturing a family, the journey becomes an opportunity for shared growth and well-being. By embracing these weight loss tips tailored to the unique challenges of parenthood, families can embark on a collective path towards health, resilience, and lasting vitality.

Weight Loss Tricks

Numerous individuals are searching for strategies to shed pounds that can assist them in their ongoing battle. Globally, people seek solutions that can distinguish between a frustrating weight loss journey and smooth, steady progress. Here are some tips crafted to aid you in discovering the right path.

Weight Loss Trick 1

If you are committed to shedding pounds, persistence is key. Great achievements require effort and the occasional sacrifice. Don't fret if it seems to be taking too long; time passes swiftly in our busy world. Utilize this time to transform into a better and healthier version of yourself.

Weight Loss Trick 2

Acknowledge and reward yourself upon reaching significant milestones. It's a proven psychological strategy to indulge in small treats as a celebration for accomplishing something meaningful. Losing your initial five kilograms is a crucial milestone, so treat yourself to a visit to your favorite restaurant. Exercise restraint while there, but revel in the satisfaction of hitting a significant target.

Weight Loss Trick 3

Incorporate plenty of salad into your diet. Salad is low in calories but rich in water and nutrients. It allows you to enjoy substantial meals without feeling hungry while reducing the intake of empty calories. This can be highly beneficial, as most people consume an excessive number of calories.

Weight Loss Trick 4

If you sweeten your tea or coffee, consider reducing the number of cups you consume. Many individuals habitually drink five or six cups of coffee or tea daily, adding unnecessary calories when sugar is included. Opt for a healthier alternative for those extra calories or eliminate them altogether to aid in your weight loss journey.

Chapter 8

Achieving Sustainable Weight Loss: The Importance of Realistic Long-Term Goals

The prevalence of weight-related concerns and body image struggles has led many individuals to seek effective weight loss methods. Amidst the plethora of resources available, the confusion surrounding which approach to adopt can be overwhelming for those grappling with excess weight. While the fundamentals of weight loss remain consistent, emphasizing realistic goals, calorie reduction, and incorporating moderate exercise is crucial. Contrary to popular belief, successful weight loss programs are grounded in rationality, flexibility, and overall health, making them accessible to anyone committed to their weight loss journey.

Setting Reachable Goals

The initial and fundamental step towards successful weight loss is establishing achievable goals. Understanding the motivation behind weight reduction, identifying the benefits anticipated upon program completion, and acknowledging the necessary dietary modifications are key aspects of goal setting. This introspection not only enhances self-awareness but also aids in establishing realistic and sustainable weight loss objectives.

It is imperative that weight loss goals are both reasonable and gradual. For instance, aiming to lose 1kg per week is a practical target. Once the goal is set, the next step involves maintaining a food journal. This journal serves as a tool for analyzing and monitoring dietary habits throughout the week. Keeping a record of consumed foods and beverages, as well as noting personal feelings toward these choices, sheds light

The Practical 30-Day Meal Plan

Day 1 Meal Plan:

Meal 1 (Breakfast)

- A Whole Egg with oatmeal and Small Glass of Skim Milk
- Snack 1 (Mid- Morning) Low Sugar Strawberry Yogurt used for dipping Banana

Meal 2 (Lunch)

- Turkey Breast with Brown Rice
- Snack 2 (Late Afternoon) Low Sugar Strawberry Yogurt used for dipping Banana

Meal 3 (Dinner)

- Grilled Tuna with Asparagus
- Snack 3 (Late Evening) Small Handful of Unsalted Walnuts on Small Salad

Day 2 Meal Plan
Meal 1 (Breakfast)

- Cream of Wheat with Glass of Skim Milk
- Snack 1 (Mid- Morning) Low- Fat Cottage Cheese with Blueberries

Meal 2 (Lunch)

- Whole Wheat wrap with Turkey and Low- Fat Cheese
- Snack 2 (Late Afternoon) Low- Fat Cottage Cheese with Blueberries

Meal 3 (Dinner)

- Baked Chicken Breast with Broccoli
- Snack 3 (Late Evening) A Low- Fat Cheese Stick with a Few Celery Sticks

Day 3 Meal Plan
Meal 1 (Breakfast)

- Oatmeal with Skim Milk
- Snack 1 (Mid- Morning) ½ Banana with Low- Fat Yogurt

Meal 2 (Lunch)

- Grilled Chicken Breast with small sweet potatoSnack 2 (Late Afternoon) Apple with ¼ handful of unsalted almonds

Meal 3 (Dinner)

- Grilled Salmon with Asparagus
- Snack 3 (Late Evening) Celery Sticks

Day 4 Meal Plan
Meal 1 (Breakfast)

- Turkey Bacon with Egg and Whole Grain Toast
- Snack 1 (Mid- Morning) Can of Tuna with Watermelon

Meal 2 (Lunch)

- Grilled Chicken on Bed of Salad Greens with Whole Grain Crackers
- Snack 2 (Late Afternoon) Mango with Low- Fat Cheese Sticks

Meal 3 (Dinner)

- Broiled Salmon with Green Salad
- Snack 3 (Late Evening) Celery Sticks w/ small Amount of Natural Peanut Butter

Day 5 Meal Plan

Meal 1 (Breakfast)

- 2 Slices of Whole Grain Bread, a Whole Egg and some Egg Whites
- Snack 1 (Mid- Morning) Peaches with Low- Sugar Yogurt

Meal 2 (Lunch)

- Sweet Potato with Broiled Turkey Burgers
- Snack 2 (Late Afternoon) Can of Tuna with Watermelon

Meal 3 (Dinner)

- Baked Tilapia with Cold Spinach Salad
- Snack 3 (Late Evening) Plain Low Fat Yogurt used as Dip for Veggie Sticks

Day 6 Meal Plan

Meal 1 (Breakfast)

- Slice of whole grain bread w/ teaspoon of peanut butter and
- Medium Glass of Low Fat or Skim Milk
- Snack 1 (Mid- Morning) Mango with Low- Fat Cheese Sticks

Meal 2 (Lunch)

- Whole Wheat Pasta with Boiled Shrimp
- Snack 2 (Late Afternoon) Bit of High Fiber Whole Grain Cereal mixed w/ low sugar applesauce + Walnuts

Meal 3 (Dinner)

- Grilled Chicken Breast with Sliced Cucumbers
- Snack 3 (Late Evening) Plain Low Fat Yogurt used as Dip for Veggie Sticks

Day 7 Meal Plan

Meal 1 (Breakfast)

- Healthy higher fiber cold cereal with low fat or Skim milk
- Snack 1 (Mid- Morning) A Couple of Low Fat Cheese Sticks and a Mango

Meal 2 (Lunch)

- Grilled Tilapia with a Small Serving of Whole Wheat Pasta
- Snack 2 (Late Afternoon) 1 Cup of Low Sugar Yogurt with Strawberries

Meal 3 (Dinner)

- Grilled Turkey Breast with Cooked Spinach with Dash of Vinegar
- Snack 3 (Late Evening) Small serving of Canned Chicken with a Sliced Cucumber

Day 8 Meal Plan

Meal 1 (Breakfast)

- Plain Oatmeal with a whole egg and some egg whites
- Snack 1 (Mid- Morning) Half a handful of unsalted almonds and a half handful of blueberries

Meal 2 (Lunch)

- Grilled Tuna Steak with a Medium Sweet Potato
- Snack 2 (Late Afternoon) Low Fat Cottage Cheese with pineapple

Meal 3 (Dinner)

- Chicken and Shrimp Stir Fry with Vegetable Medley
- Snack 3 (Late Evening) A Small Can of Tuna with some Raw Veggies

Day 9 Meal Plan

Meal 1 (Breakfast)

- Whole Wheat Wrap with Peanut Butter and Small Glass of Skim Milk
- Snack 1 (Mid- Morning) Half a handful of unsalted almonds and small apple

Meal 2 (Lunch)

- 1 Peanut Butter sandwich on whole grain bread
- Snack 2 (Late Afternoon) 1 cup of lower sugar yogurt with a peach

Meal 3 (Dinner)

- Grilled Turkey Burgers with Grilled Veggie Kabobs
- Snack 3 (Late Evening) A Low Fat Cheese Stick with some Cucumber Slices

Day 10 Meal Plan

Meal 1 (Breakfast)

- Healthy higher fiber cold cereal with low fat or Skim milk
- Snack 1 (Mid- Morning) 1 cup of lower sugar yogurt with a banana

Meal 2 (Lunch)

- 1 turkey sandwich (lots of turkey) with low fat cheese on whole grain bread
- Snack 2 (Late Afternoon) Half a handful of unsalted almonds and small pear

Meal 3 (Dinner)

- Grilled Turkey Burgers with Grilled Veggie Kabobs
- Snack 3 (Late Evening) Celery Sticks with a small spread of Peanut Butter

Day 11 Meal Plan

Meal 1 (Breakfast)

- 1 Whole Egg, ½ Chicken Breast, and 1 Slice of Whole Grain Bread
- Snack 1 (Mid- Morning) Unsalted Almonds with Pear

Meal 2 (Lunch)

- 1 chicken breast sandwich on whole wheat/grain w/ mustard and w/ out mayo
- Snack 2 (Late Afternoon) Apple Slices with teaspoon Peanut Butter

Meal 3 (Dinner)

- Grilled Halibut with Cooked Zucchini and Yellow Squash
- Snack 3 (Late Evening) Celery Sticks with Plain low- sugar yogurt for dipping

Day 12 Meal Plan

Meal 1 (Breakfast)

- Cream of Wheat with 1 Whole Egg
- Snack 1 (Mid- Morning) Walnuts (Unsalted) with an Orange

Meal 2 (Lunch)

- Mozzarella and tomato sandwich (Whole wheat or grain)
- Snack 2 (Late Afternoon) Half a handful of Unsalted Pecans and a half handful of Cherries

Meal 3 (Dinner)

- Lean grilled pork chops w/ green beans
- Snack 3 (Late Evening) Cucumber Sticks w/ plain Yogurt for Dipping

Day 13 Meal Plan

Meal 1 (Breakfast)

- Oatmeal with Turkey Bacon small glass of Skim Milk
- Snack 1 (Mid- Morning) ½ Handful Unsalted Almonds with Pear

Meal 2 (Lunch)

- Peanut butter and banana sandwich on whole wheat or grain bread
- Snack 2 (Late Afternoon) Half a handful of unsalted Pecans and an Orange

Meal 3 (Dinner)

- Grilled chicken breast and asparagus
- Snack 3 (Late Evening) Raw Cauliflower Sticks w/teaspoon of low fat Dip

Day 14 Meal Plan

Meal 1 (Breakfast)

- Healthy higher fiber cold cereal with low fat or Skim milk
- Snack 1 (Mid- Morning) A Couple of Low Fat Cheese Sticks and a large Orange

Meal 2 (Lunch)

- **1** Tablespoon Almond Butter on whole grain or wheat crackers
- Snack 2 (Late Afternoon) Low Fat Cottage Cheese with a small Papaya

Meal 3 (Dinner)

- Unsalted Pecans on Green Salad with Oil and Vinegar Dressing
- Snack 3 (Late Evening) Raw Broccoli Sticks w/teaspoon of low fat Dip

Day 15 Meal Plan
Meal 1 (Breakfast)

- A Whole Grain English Muffin w/ slice of low- fat cheese and Small
- Glass of Skim Milk
- Snack 1 (Mid- Morning) A Peach and a large teaspoon scoop of Peanut Butter

Meal 2 (Lunch)

- Black Beans and Rice (brown or wild rice)
- Snack 2 (Late Afternoon) Low Sugar Plain Yogurt used for dipping Peach Slices

Meal 3 (Dinner)

- Grilled Shrimp with Asparagus and Mushrooms
- Snack 3 (Late Evening) Small Handful of Unsalted Pecans on Small Salad

Day 16 Meal Plan

Meal 1 (Breakfast)

- A Whole Grain English Muffin w/ peanut butter spread and Small
- Glass of Skim Milk
- Snack 1 (Mid- Morning) Apple Slices with Almond Butter spread

Meal 2 (Lunch)

- Red Beans and Rice (brown or wild rice)
- Snack 2 (Late Afternoon) Low Sugar Plain Yogurt used for dipping Apple Slices

Meal 3 (Dinner)

- Baked Scallops with Cabbage
- Snack 3 (Late Evening) Small Handful of Unsalted Walnuts on Small Salad

Day 17 Meal Plan
Meal 1 (Breakfast)

- A Bran Cereal w/ Skim Milk
- Snack 1 (Mid- Morning) Pineapple with Low Fat Cottage Cheese

Meal 2 (Lunch)

- Pinto Beans and 2 Slices Whole Grain Toast
- Snack 2 (Late Afternoon) Low Sugar Blueberry Yogurt and a Plum

Meal 3 (Dinner)

- Grilled Grouper with Fresh Onion, Cucumber, and Tomato Slices
- Snack 3 (Late Evening) Small Low Sugar Yogurt and Celery Sticks

Day 18 Meal Plan

Meal 1 (Breakfast)

- Puffed Wheat Cereal w/ Skim Milk
- Snack 1 (Mid- Morning) Mandarin Orange w/ large teaspoon scoop of Almond Butter

Meal 2 (Lunch)

- No Skin Cornish Hen with Sweet Potato
- Snack 2 (Late Afternoon) Nectarine w/ strawberry yogurt

Meal 3 (Dinner)

- Small Filet Mignon w/ Mushrooms and Cold Spinach Salad
- Snack 3 (Late Evening) Fresh Carrot Sticks w/ Plain Yogurt Dip

Day 19 Meal Plan
Meal 1 (Breakfast)

- Shredded Wheat Cereal w/ Skim Milk
- Snack 1 (Mid- Morning) Nectarine w/ large teaspoon scoop of Peanut Butter

Meal 2 (Lunch)

- No Skin, White Meat Rotisserie Chicken w/ Brown Rice
- Snack 2 (Late Afternoon) Mandarin Orange w/ blueberry yogurt

Meal 3 (Dinner)

- Lean Flank Steak w/ Cooked Summer Squash and Zucchini
- Snack 3 (Late Evening) Fresh Broccoli Sticks with Plain Yogurt Dip

Day 20 Meal Plan

Meal 1 (Breakfast)

- Whole Grain Waffles with Turkey Bacon and a Glass of Skim Milk
- Snack 1 (Mid- Morning) Handful of Blackberries and Vanilla Yogurt

Meal 2 (Lunch)

- Green Salad w/ Egg Whites, Cucumbers, & Tomatoes & Whole Wheat
- Crackers plus Olive Oil and Vinegar Based Dressing
- Snack 2 (Late Afternoon) A Pear and a Handful of Almonds

Meal 3 (Dinner)

- Turkey Sausage (low sodium) with Sauerkraut
- Snack 3 (Late Evening) Cucumber Slices w/ hot sauce and a few Unsalted Walnuts

Day 21 Meal Plan
Meal 1 (Breakfast)

- High Fiber Cereal with Skim Milk
- Snack 1 (Mid- Morning) Handful of Blueberries and Plain Yogurt

Meal 2 (Lunch)

- Green Salad w/ Almonds, Cucumbers, & Tomatoes & Whole Wheat Crackers plus Olive Oil and Vinegar Based Dressing
- Snack 2 (Late Afternoon) Low Fat Yogurt and Papaya

Meal 3 (Dinner)

- Chicken Sausage (low sodium) with Sauerkraut
- Snack 3 (Late Evening) Cucumber Slices w/a few Unsalted Almonds

Day 22 Meal Plan

Meal 1 (Breakfast)

- 1 Egg Yolk and 2 Egg Whites w Whole Grain Toast
- Snack 1 (Mid- Morning) Handful of Strawberries and Vanilla Yogurt

Meal 2 (Lunch)

- Green Salad w/ Pecans, Cucumbers, & Tomatoes & Whole Wheat
- Crackers plus Olive Oil and Vinegar Based Dressing
- Snack 2 (Late Afternoon) 2 Plums with a Small Handful of Pecans

Meal 3 (Dinner)

- Kidney Beans w/ Grilled Eggplant and Fresh Tomato Slices
- Snack 3 (Late Evening) Cucumber Slices w/a few Unsalted Pecans

Day 23 Meal Plan

Meal 1 (Breakfast)

- Kashi Cereal with Low Fat or Skim Milk
- Snack 1 (Mid- Morning) Handful of Cherries and Plain Yogurt

Meal 2 (Lunch)

- Grilled Chicken Breast on a Green Salad w/ Oil & Vinegar Dressing
- Snack 2 (Late Afternoon) Apple w/ Peanut Butter

Meal 3 (Dinner)

- Eggs and Fresh Salsa with Sliced Cucumbers
- Snack 3 (Late Evening) Veggie Sticks and Low Fat Yogurt

Day 24 Meal Plan

Meal 1 (Breakfast)

- Turkey Bacon, Whole Grain Toast and a Glass of Skim Milk
- Snack 1 (Mid- Morning) Handful of Unsalted Almonds and 1/2 Handful of Fresh Strawberries

Meal 2 (Lunch)

- Grilled Turkey Burgers w/ Brown Rice
- Snack 2 (Late Afternoon) Mango Slices and ½ handful of Peanuts

Meal 3 (Dinner)

- Homemade Chicken and Vegetable Soup
- Snack 3 (Late Evening) Cucumber Slices w/ hot sauce w/ small handful of Pecans

Day 25 Meal Plan

Meal 1 (Breakfast)

- Whole Egg w/ Egg Whites and a Whole Grain Waffle
- Snack 1 (Mid- Morning) Low Fat Cottage Cheese with Peaches

Meal 2 (Lunch)

- Chicken Fajitas w/ Corn or Whole Wheat Tortillas w/ Wild Rice
- Snack 2 (Late Afternoon) ½ Handful of Walnuts w/ an Orange

Meal 3 (Dinner)

- Homemade Turkey and Vegetable Soup
- Snack 3 (Late Evening) Low Fat Yogurt used for Dipping Veggie Sticks

Day 26 Meal Plan

Meal 1 (Breakfast)

- Plain Oatmeal and one Slice of Whole Grain Toast w/teaspoon of peanut butter
- Snack 1 (Mid- Morning) Low Fat Cheese Stick and Papaya

Meal 2 (Lunch)

- Grilled Fish with Sweet Potato
- Snack 2 (Late Afternoon) 1 Cup of Low Sugar Yogurt with Kiwi

Meal 3 (Dinner)

- Baked Chicken with Steamed Asparagus
- Snack 3 (Late Evening) Small Green Salad w/ Small handful of Walnuts

Day 27 Meal Plan

Meal 1 (Breakfast)

- Cream of Wheat, Multi Grain Toast and Small Glass of Skim Milk
- Snack 1 (Mid- Morning) ½ Handful of Peanuts and Mandarin Oranges

Meal 2 (Lunch)

- Whole Wheat Turkey Wrap w/ Oil & Vinegar Based Dressing
- Snack 2 (Late Afternoon) Watermelon

Meal 3 (Dinner)

- Green Salad w/ Grilled Chicken Breast and Oil & Vinegar Dressing
- Snack 3 (Late Evening) 1 Cup of Low Fat Blueberry Yogurt w/ small green salad

Day 28 Meal Plan
Meal 1 (Breakfast)

- Whole Grain English Muffin w/ Low Fat Cheese and Small Glass of Skim Milk
- Snack 1 (Mid- Morning) Low Fat Cottage Cheese w/ Blueberries

Meal 2 (Lunch)

- Peanut Butter Sandwich on Whole Grain Bread
- Snack 2 (Late Afternoon) Banana Slices w/ Peanut Butter

Meal 3 (Dinner)

- Lean Grilled Pork Chops with Grilled Squash and Zucchini
- Snack 3 (Late Evening) Cucumber Slices w/ Low Fat Yogurt Used for Dipping

Day 29 Meal Plan

Meal 1 (Breakfast)

- Unsweetened Natural Granola w/ Skim Milk
- Snack 1 (Mid- Morning) Strawberries and ½ Handful of Almonds

Meal 2 (Lunch)

- Kashi Bar with Yogurt
- Snack 2 (Late Afternoon) Pear Slices with Peanut Butter spread

Meal 3 (Dinner)

- Spinach Salad w/ Oil & Vinegar Based Dressing w/ Broiled Turkey Burgers
- Snack 3 (Late Evening) 1 Cup of LowFat Plain Yogurt w/ cold raw carrots

Day 30 Meal Plan
Meal 1 (Breakfast)

- Cream of Wheat and Turkey Bacon
- Snack 1 (Mid- Morning) Papaya and 1 Low Fat Cheese Stick

Meal 2 (Lunch)

- Chicken Fajitas and Small Green Salad with corn or whole wheat tortillas
- Snack 2 (Late Afternoon) Grapes &½ Handful of Walnuts

Meal 3 (Dinner)

- Grilled Salmon w/Steamed Vegetable Medley
- Snack 3 (Late Evening) Veggie Sticks w/ Low Fat Yogurt

Conclusion

In conclusion, it would be very pertinent to say that this book isn't just about losing weight; it's about changing your mindset, emotions and habits towards food. This has to do with making friends with food and as well finding a way to stay healthy that makes sense to you. As you've followed along, I'm very sure you noticed less stress about food, a break from using it to feel better and a way of eating that fits your body.

This book is a friendly guide, showing you realistic ways to make lasting changes in your weight loss journey. Take the tips and ideas it offers and see how you can live peacefully with foods that used to tempt you.